Reiki Healing for Beginners:

101 Things You Need to Know About Reiki to Help You Discover the Power of Healing and the Peace That Exists in the Palm of Your Hands.

- Ella Hughes-

Table Of Contents

Introduction

We've all felt it before - the stress, the tiredness, the persistent feeling of unwell that seems to stem from nowhere. We try to take our minds off of the feeling, rest it off, or even pop pills to address the symptoms. But no matter what we try, we can never truly feel *free* from the discomfort and dissatisfaction.

Sound familiar?

Ask anyone when was the last time they felt completely *free* from stress, pain, and discomfort, and you're likely to hear them say it was a *long, long time ago*. That's because the fast-paced lives we lead - full of responsibilities, obligations, and expectations - make it difficult to achieve balance.

With a limited amount of energy running through our system, we end up spreading ourselves so thinly over far too many tasks than we can actually handle. In the end, we push our body to do more, to take more, and to spend more in an effort to see everything through.

Over time, this unhealthy practice of pushing our bodies to the limit can lead to a perpetual state of fatigue and dissatisfaction. We start to lose motivation, ambition, and might even start to feel *physically unwell* with illness becoming a mainstay in our lives.

But what is there for us to do? Life is hard, and these responsibilities can't wait. While it is true that there is no such thing as putting life on hold, there are things you can do to proactively rise through the challenges and become better equipped to face the difficulties thrown your way. It all lies in how well you're able to maximize the energy you have.

Ancient mystics believed that energy is a *finite* force that exists in each one of us. Unlike the common notion that energy is gained from or spent on external substances and factors like food, rest, and work, mystic healers believe that energy *can't* be used, spent, lost, or acquired.

Instead, we all have a fixed amount of energy coursing through our bodies. When we feel tired, unwell, or weak, it's not because we've *lost energy*, but because the flow of our energy has been impeded. Thus, maximizing the use of our energy depends on how well we *optimize* how it courses through our body. Unimpeded, free-flowing, well-distributed energy is what characterizes good health and optimal wellness.

If you've tried every trick in the book, yet still suffer from fatigue and a persistent feeling of unwell, then maybe it's time you tried to attune yourself to your energy. In this comprehensive guide, you'll learn everything you need to know about the effects of **reiki healing** and how you can use it to improve your quality of life.

Discover the intricacies of this mystical yet potent art form and learn the different ways it can help you achieve peak physical, emotional, and mental wellness through its simple, subtle, and effective healing techniques.

Because the answer to supreme health and wellness is in the palm of your hands.

Chapter 1:
The History and Foundation of Reiki Healing

Reiki Healing is an old spiritual healing art that started in the late 1800s. The method aims to optimize an individual's *energy flow* in order to heal a diverse range of ailments that may involve a person's physical, psychological, emotional, and even sexual health.

The centuries old practice was developed in Japan by Dr. Mikao Usui. Today, it's used as a potent healing therapy across the globe, leading people towards achieving their peak health and wellness.

1ˢᵗ *Thing you need to know...*
Dr. Usui's Spiritual Awakening

Dr. Mikao Usui was born to a wealthy Buddhist family in 1865. His parents valued education, and saw to it that their children would receive the best education available during their time. Usui was thus sent to a Buddhist monastery in his younger years where he would learn swordsmanship, martial arts, and Kiko - the Japanese version of chi kung.

As an adult, Usui spent most of his time travelling the world, learning about the unique spiritual healing practices that different countries would use to heal their sick. When he finally decided to reside in a Buddhist monastery in his home town, Usui felt a greater power calling him to connect with the universe and establish a new healing art.

During his Buddhist training, Usui traveled to Mount Kurama where he would spend the next 21 days in deep meditation. He fasted and prayed for three weeks, and on the last day of his practice, he experienced spiritual awakening.

He opened his eyes and saw Sanskrit symbols flash before him. As he made sense of the otherworldly information, he developed the Reiki healing method, which is what he would impart to 2,000 others throughout the remainder of his lifetime.

In 1922, Usui founded the first Reiki clinic and school where he would train thousands of students in the art form he had discovered during his meditation. One of these students would be Dr. Chujiro Hayashi.

2nd *Thing you need to know...*

Dr. Chujiro Hayashi's Role in Spreading Reiki

Chujiro Hayashi was one of Usui's best students, and he went on to establish his own reiki healing clinic in Tokyo. But more than simply following Dr. Usui's original method, Hayashi sought to improve the art and add more techniques in order to achieve full body healing.

Dr. Hayashi took his version of reiki healing and went on to teach more students and turn them into reiki healing masters. One of those students - Mrs. Hawayo Takata - studied the process and took her learning to the United States, which marked the spread of reiki healing throughout the western world.

3rd *Thing you need to know...*

Reiki Healing Addresses the Self First

One of the foundations of Dr. Usui's principles is that reiki healing aims to *heal the self first*. As a healing practice, reiki works by honing your healing energy in order to repair flaws in another person's energy flow. If the healer himself has problems with his energy, then it is very possible to pass these irregularities to the person being healed.

That said, one of the major facets of reiki healing is to first target the self with healing energy. That's where the genius of the reiki healing practice lies - that it can be used to heal your own energy problems, allowing you to establish a deeper, richer relationship with yourself in order to attain the highest level of wellness and health possible.

4th *Thing you need to know...*

Reiki Healing Does Not Tie In With a Specific Religion

Other healing methods that come from the East are closely tied with religious practices. For instance, Yoga has been known to work closely with principles from the Buddhist and Hindu belief systems. Of course, that doesn't dampen the benefits of Yoga, but because of these ties, it might be difficult for individuals outside of that belief system to fully understand and grasp the practice of Yoga.

That's why reiki healing has adapted so well as a healing method all around the world. Without having any ties to specific religious practices or belief systems, reiki transcends some of the most common barriers that people face. Thus, the technique can be easily adapted by anyone without having to deal with contradictions to their beliefs and religious practices.

5th *Thing you need to know...*

Reiki is a Holistic Healing Method

The beauty of reiki as a healing method is that it's a holistic treatment technique that targets anything and everything that you might be dealing with. The basic idea of reiki is that *energy* - the life force in our bodies - is what drives all of the different aspects of our being. From our physical health, to our emotional, mental, and sexual health, this life force is what our bodies use to achieve all the different processes that make us human.

With this basic principle, reiki becomes a holistic healing method because it targets disturbances in our energy flow which can have a direct impact on the different facets of our health. By targeting specific energy centers, reiki aims to heal a spectrum of conditions - from those that can be physically felt, to those that might be more insidious in nature.

6th *Thing you need to know...*

Anyone Can Be a Reiki Healer

Perhaps the most promising aspect of reiki healing is that it's something *anyone can learn*. Reiki doesn't require healers to have any sort of religious, educational, or cultural background, thus making it a healing practice for anyone and everyone.

The only things that learners really need in their effort to discover the truth of reiki healing is the willingness to learn and hone their skills. So, if you feel you're ready to unlock the powerful healing capabilities of reiki, then it's time to learn the basics.

Chapter 2:
Reiki Healing For
Holistic Health

How can you benefit from reiki healing? Some people think that the process of reiki healing is strictly spiritual, but that isn't actually the case. This ancient Japanese healing art is utilized for the entire spectrum of human conditions - from those involving your physical body, to those that manifest in more subtle ways, like psychological or emotional stress and illness.

Reiki healing can target almost anything that afflicts your system and compromises your health - regardless of what plane of your being that disturbance exists.

7th *Thing you need to know...*

Understanding How Life Force Works

To better understand how reiki works, it's important to first understand the life force that it targets. Your *life force* can be likened to your blood - free flowing and abundant, passing through every inch of your body. Unlike your blood however, your life force *can't* be reduced, lost, or replaced. Even in the presence of injury - such as cuts or open wounds - you will *not lose energy*.

Instead, energy becomes *blocked* whenever you're injured, sick, or unwell. For example, if you fracture a limb, the energy in that specific area of your body is impeded. In effect, you feel pain, discomfort, and your immunity is reduced, putting your body at risk of infection.

The principle works the same way for your psychological, emotional, and even your sexual well-being. Any sort of disturbance in these aspects of your life can result to a blockage in the flow of your life force.

Reiki healing aims to restore the proper flow of this energy by removing blockages and improving the way that the energy flows throughout your system. In effect, reiki can address the different areas of your body - whether physical or cognitive - and eliminate the blockages that exist therein.

8th *Thing you need to know...*

The Role of Stress

The biggest insult to your life force is stress. The more stressed you feel, the lower your immunity gets. Stress comes from a variety of sources - from your daily interactions, to your responsibilities and work, and everything in between.

That's why if you take the time to consider the principles of reiki meditation (discussed in the next chapter), most of the points actually address potential stressors you experience day to day.

Aside from targeting illness, disease, and blockages in your life force, reiki also aims to reduce the amount of stress you feel. At the end of each healing session, you should feel a renewed sense of peace and calm, making you far less prone to the pressure and negative emotions that situations around you might evoke.

With increased resistance and resilience against stress, you can curb a diverse range of conditions and even ease away the symptoms of the problems you currently face.

9ᵗʰ Thing you need to know...
Reiki Accelerates Healing

Not a lot of people believe that reiki can be an effective method for *physical healing*. Essentially, physical healing involves restoring wellness especially where injury, disease, or illness might be present. These include conditions that afflict the different organ systems and body parts that make up our being.

When your body experiences physical injury or disease, your life force flows much more slowly, especially where the injury exists. Think of it like a damaged highway, where roadworks prevent traffic from progressing freely. Cars pile up and traffic slows down, creating a stressful situation that causes a variety of negative emotions to arise.

In the same way, blocked energy can create stress and limit your body's immune response. By way of reiki, repair can be accelerated, making it possible for you to enjoy renewed health and well-being sooner rather than later.

10th *Thing you need to know...*

Reiki Assists in Detox

Each one of us has an accumulation of toxins that we take in from the environment around us. From the food we eat to the air we breathe, these toxins exist by the millions, and we come into contact with them every day. With extended exposure, toxins overload our system. That's why you might experience things like acne, blemishes, tiredness, illness, and stress.

One of the benefits of reiki is that it removes toxins from the body. Optimizing the flow of life force clears away the toxins that might have built up in your system, allowing energy to flow more freely. On top of that, cleansing away toxins also improves your positive energy.

11ᵗʰ *Thing you need to know...*

Reiki Helps You Discover the Healer Within

It's somewhat ironic how reiki works. Everyone has an *inner healer* that they might not fully know. Reiki helps you establish a connection with this inner healer so that you can discover new ways to optimize your own health. But to perform reiki healing, you have to first tap into your inner healing potential.

All things considered, it's easy to see that reiki is a healing art that's perfected with practice and time. The more you try your capabilities, the deeper your understanding of reiki becomes. Fortunately, there is no *wrong way* to try to tap into your healing potential as long as you focus on positivity.

Always start with the reiki meditation process first to be able to optimize your healing energy. The more you try the process, the better the benefits will become over time. With enough practice, you might even be able to heal others around you as you discover how to *feel* energy and determine where illness and blockages might lie.

12^(th) *Thing you need to know...*

Reiki Improves Your Immune Response

The more stressed your system is, the more prone it becomes to illness and disease. Keep in mind that the flow of your life force can be slowed down when you're subjected to too much stress and pressure. And when the flow is slow, impeded, or blocked, then the efficiency of your energy becomes limited.

Life energy is an essential factor in a variety of biological and physiological processes. Therefore, when the flow slows down, our bodies become prone to disease. With reiki, energy can be optimized to flow at the right speed and with enough vigor. In doing so, we can improve our immune response and protect our system from potential threats.

13th *Thing you need to know...*

Reiki Can Heal Almost Anything

What can reiki heal? In a nutshell, reiki can heal almost anything. Targeting your energy flow, reiki aims to restore optimal health by influencing energy in your system to relieve illness. Perhaps the only time that reiki can't heal a person is if they aren't fully dedicated to the process. Otherwise, reiki can be exceptionally beneficial for overall wellness.

Can reiki heal you to full well-being? That depends. There are some conditions that might not be fully addressed. For instance, with chronic conditions like diabetes when the damage to your system might be deeply ingrained, reiki healing might not be able to bring full healing. That's especially true if there are a variety of other factors that compound your condition, like your lifestyle, diet, and genetic predisposition.

Nonetheless, reiki healing can be particularly beneficial because it still optimizes energy flow, bestowing wellness and positivity where it can in order to reduce the symptoms of your condition.

Chapter 3:
The Intricacies of
Intention Setting

Much like other ancient healing techniques, so too does reiki follow a systematic flow of steps. This pattern helps make sure that you're prepared and well-equipped throughout the entire process, guaranteeing that your mindset is appropriate and that your energy is as positive as it can be.

Just like crystal healing, the process of reiki healing also begins with an integral first step - *setting your intention*

14th Thing you need to know...
The Importance of Breaking Self Limits

Before any healing practice takes place, it's vital that you break any limitations you might have imposed on yourself or your healing capabilities. First time healers will often struggle with this, thinking that they're not *prepared or good enough* to heal themselves through reiki.

Self-doubt can be a powerful mechanism that works against your real potential. Therefore, it's best that you work away these limitations first before you engage in healing to maximize the benefits of your practice.

While it's normal for you to feel apprehensive about your capacity to heal yourself, there are things you can do to feel more confident and capable in your reiki healing power. The best way would be to *write affirmations* that reduce your self doubt and make you more trusting of the process you're about to undertake.

As the first step of your healing, take a piece of paper and a pen, and write down affirmations that make you feel more trusting of your inherent healing power. Here are some examples of affirmations that you can write down:

- *I am an empowered, capable child of the divine universe. I am deserving of all the positivity that life has to offer.*

- *My heartfelt desires deserve to be fulfilled.*

- *I am open to the gifts of the universe. My arms are spread wide to receive all the positivity that comes my way. I am receptive of these gifts and blessings.*

- *I am capable of healing. I have the power inside of me, and this potent gift cannot be corrupted - only improved and enhanced.*

As you write your affirmation, make sure to truly feel the meaning of the words. Meditate upon the words and feel the energy of the universe flowing into your system. Visualize the benefits of reiki healing and try to picture out your life after you've received these gifts. Strive to become the person in your visions and choose to trust in your inherent ability to become your own healer.

15th *Thing you need to know...*

Setting Your Intention

Once you feel more confident in your healing capabilities, it's time to set your intention. Your intention is basically what you want to achieve with your reiki healing practice. There is no wrong or right way to state your intention, and there is no aspect of your being that can't be made an intention. So essentially, whatever it is you feel needs healing can be set as your intention to maximize the benefits of your reiki healing practice.

Throughout the day, you probably already set intentions in some shape, way, or form. *"I hope I can finish my workload today. I wish my mom takes my pregnancy news positively. I pray my boss agrees to my request for a raise."* All of these statements demonstrate intentions that we set for ourselves in our daily lives.

In the same way, your reiki healing intention is what you *aim to achieve* through the healing practice. By setting your intention, you can direct your effort more specifically in order to restore the flow of your life force where you might be experiencing disturbance.

16th Thing you need to know...

Specific Intentions are More Effective

The more specific you are when it comes to setting your intentions, the more effective your healing practice becomes. *Why?* Remember that the process of directing the healing energy where you want it to go will rely on your own capabilities. The more specific your intention, the more precisely you'll be able to direct the healing power to achieve the results you want.

For instance, instead of saying *"I want to be pregnant someday",* opt for something more specific, like *"I will conceive by June of this year and have a healthy baby boy by March of next year."*

See how it changes the energy of your intention? By being as specific as possible, it becomes easier to visualize the fruit of your reiki healing practice. And in effect, you become more capable of directing your healing energy where it needs to be for a more effective effort.

17th Thing you need to know...

Positive Intentions are Best

It's always easier to mention all the things you don't want. But by phrasing your intention in a negative way, you might also have a negative impact on the positivity of the energy you imbibe. Negative intentions create an atmosphere of dislike, dissatisfaction, and unhappiness, which may stir negative emotions as you go through the healing process.

Avoid using negative words like "don't", "won't", and "can't", and focus on more positive versions of your intentions in order to reap the maximum benefits of your healing practice. For instance, instead of saying "*I won't fall victim to the same emotional stress that my ex put me through*", opt for something more positive like, "*I will discover a genuine, pure love that will bring me greater joy and satisfaction than I've ever known.*"

18th *Thing you need to know...*

Always Strive for the Most

Your intention doesn't simply end with what you want for yourself. In most instances, the universe will surprise you by giving you things that exceed your own expectations. So, don't limit your intentions by adding finality. Instead, add a phrase at the end of each intention in order to maximize the potential rewards of your healing practice.

How do you do this? Adding phrases like "... or better" or "...or more" can be simple yet powerful ways to increase the potential of your intention. So, for instance, using the previous example, you might say something like "*I will discover a genuine, pure love that will bring me greater joy and satisfaction than I've ever known or better.*"

19th *Thing you need to know...*

Keep It Personal

Personal intentions work best because the only person you truly know is yourself. We can't control other people's fate, and neither are we responsible for other people's wellness. Only they will understand what they want and need in life, so it's best that you keep other people out of your intentions.

For instance, a mother might say *"I want my daughter to become the best in her class."* But because her daughter's energy is disconnected from her own life force system, it might be impossible to achieve that intention.

Instead, try to focus on yourself and what you can do to have a positive impact on other people in your life. For instance, the above intention can be rephrased to *"I will become a supportive, understanding, and empathetic mother so that my daughter will have the guidance and love she needs in order to succeed."*

If you're trying to heal someone else with your energy, avoid setting intentions for them. Instead, give them the basic principles of proper intention setting and then ask them to formulate their own intention.

20th Thing you need to know...

The Process of Setting

Now that you know the intention you want to work with, it's time that you actually set the intention. So how do you do that? For some, more experienced reiki healers who are attuned with their healing power, simply uttering the intention like a mantra during meditation can be more than enough for them to be able to direct their energy.

But if you're just starting out, then you might want to consider writing your intention down. There is a unique power to writing an intention, making it easier to visualize your end goal. As a beginner, it works best to write your intention on a slip of paper before starting the healing process in order to better focus your energy and achieve the results you're aiming for.

Take a clean sheet of paper and meditate on the intention you want to focus on. Once you've decided on how best to phrase your intention, write it down on your paper while wording it out. After you've written it, take the paper in your hands and read the intention a few times to yourself until it feels like you've fully absorbed its essence.

As you read your intention, visualize the energy of reiki flowing from the environment around you, towards the words on the paper. Charge your intention and sense the power of reiki blessing the words you've written.

Now that the intention is fully realized and properly set, you can begin the process of healing.

Chapter 4:
Meditation in
Preparation for
Healing

When Dr. Usui developed his reiki healing practice, he highlighted 5 different principles to guide his learners towards achieving the proper healing technique. These principles come together to form *Hatsurei-Ho* - otherwise known as reiki guided meditation. The purpose of the practice is to focus the healers mind and to open their body to the positive impact that reiki can have on their life force.

Before starting off any reiki healing session - whether on yourself or on anyone else - it's important to start with guided meditation first. This removes any impurities from your energy, improving the flow of your life force and heightening positive energy for a more enriching, effective healing experience.

21st *Thing you need to know...*

Understanding the Phrasing for Reiki Principles

One thing you'll notice about each reiki meditation principle is that they're all preceded by the phrase "just for today." Before you engage in meditation, it's important to understand *why that specific phrase is an important part of the entire principle*.

There are lots of meditation practices out there that encourage you to formulate impossible promises to yourself and to others around you, that might not actually be doable. In effect, you feel guilty and unhappy when you fail to meet the promises you made during your meditation practice.

That's why the reiki healing meditation practice encourages you to start each principle with *"just for today."* The practice understands that not everyone can experience a flawless flow of energy every day for their entire lives. Disturbances to your life force - whether in the form of illness or emotional baggage or anything in between - can and will happen somewhere down the line.

The objective of the reiki meditation practice is not to pressure you into adhering to your promises or to formulate unrealistic goals that you might not reach. Instead, it understands that guidance and healing is something that we all need *on a daily basis*. So, if for some reason, you find that today doesn't work out in your favor, there will always be tomorrow.

Once you're able to fully understand the way that these principles are phrased, then you can experience the complete benefits of the guided meditation practice.

22nd *Thing you need to know...*

Just for Today, I Will Not Worry

The first principle in the reiki meditation practice is "*just for today, I will not worry.*" As the first principle, it does hold significant importance compared to some of the others on the list. The basic idea is that *worry* uses your positive energy and converts it to negativity. When you spend your time thinking too much about future events, you'll find that it will impact your entire life negatively.

Instead of focusing on negativities and worrying about things that you can't completely predict, approach situations with a positive, can-do attitude. Assess what you're worrying about. Can you change it? Can you do something about it? If you answered yes, then that's precisely what you should do. If you answered no, then there's no need to worry.

23ʳᵈ *Thing you need to know...*

Just for Today, I Will Not Be Angry

Anger is one of the strongest emotions people feel. And as you would have expected, it's also responsible for a lot of the stress and negativity we feel. While anger is an appropriate response to a variety of situations, there is a limit as to the extent of anger that's healthy for *you*.

If you allow anger to transform your energy and limit your positivity, you will experience its negative impacts on your life force. What's more, anger that's not resolved will come back in uglier ways later on. That's why it's important to make sure that you avoid anger at all costs.

The second principle of the reiki meditation process encourages practitioners to refuse anger. There are better, more tactful ways to address frustrating situations. Be one step ahead of yourself at all times and make a firm resolve to refuse the negative impact of anger on your wellness.

Remember - your objective isn't to preserve the feelings of the person who wronged you, but to preserve your own positive energy.

24th *Thing you need to know...*

Just for Today, I Will Do My Work Honestly

You are naturally gifted and talented, with abilities that are beneficial not only to yourself, but to others around you. When you perform your work with the basic intention of just 'getting it over with', you cheat others and yourself because you're capable of much, much more.

As the third principle for reiki meditation, the goal of doing your work honestly is to perform your tasks *to the best of your abilities* and not just because you want to get them done. Offer up your best and be honest in all that you do - you'll give justice to your natural talents and gifts, and enrich your energy and life force along the way.

25th *Thing you need to know...*

Just for Today, I Will Be Thankful for My Blessings

When was the last time you took a step back to look at all the different ways that you've been blessed? All too often, we focus on the negative things in our lives. Plans that don't go our way, overdue bills, angry bosses and difficult coworkers - it's easy to see all the different aspects of our lives that might not be what we want them to.

But maintaining your attention on these negative events can cause bad energy to thrive in your system. The foundation of a positive outlook is an awareness of the many wonderful blessings that you have in your life. The more readily you're able to pick out these blessings, the stronger your positivity becomes.

26th *Thing you need to know...*

Just for Today, I Will Be Kind to My Neighbor and All Living Things

These days, it's easy to lose track of all the other living creatures around us. As the 'selfie' generation, we tend to put ourselves as the center of our lives, creating a negative, 'every-man-for-himself' mentality. But the change starts with you.

As part of your meditation practice, keep your neighbor and the other wonderful creatures of the world in mind. Acknowledge that their experiences are real and valid, and that they are equally as important as you are. The more you value the lives of others around you, the easier it becomes for you to appreciate anything and everything that happens around you.

27th *Thing you need to know...*

Hasturei-Ho Follows a Process

The Hatsurei-Ho practice follows a specific,

guided process in order to help healers cleanse their energy and prepare for the reiki healing technique. By following this structured method, you open up the opportunity to perform reiki healing with optimized life force flowing through your system.

28th Thing you need to know...

The First Step: Seiza

Start off in a comfortable seated position with the legs tucked under the body. An alternative pose would be to sit up straight in a chair.

29th Thing you need to know...

The Second Step: Mokuken

In a state of mindfulness, mention the intention "I'm beginning Hatsurie-Ho." During this time, you can start meditating on the five principles mentioned above. Keep in mind that your objective is to *cleanse your life force*.

30th Thing you need to know...
The Third Step: Kenyoku

At this point, you will start the process of dry bathing. The objective of this step is to cleanse the body and remove any impurities by using the clean, positive energy around you.

- Position your right hand over your left shoulder, and then swipe diagonally downwards. Do the same with your opposite hand and shoulder.

- Open your right palm and extend your arm. Your hand should be parallel with the floor, with your palm facing upwards.

- Position your left hand over your right shoulder and move your hand over the length of your right arm towards your open palm. Envision the negativity in your system being swept away and collected into your palm during the process.

- Repeat the previous step using your opposite hand and arm.

31st *Thing you need to know...*

The Fourth Step: Joshin Kokyu Ho

This breathing technique spreads positive life force throughout your body. Breathe in deeply through your nose, and visualize the energy flowing through your nostrils all the way to your root chakra. Exhale out involving your entire being in the process. Repeat the breathing slowly and deliberately for at least 10 minutes, aiming to live in the *now*.

32nd *Thing you need to know...*

The Fifth Step: Gassho

During this phase, your objective is to localize your energy into a single focal point. Press your palms together and focus on your middle fingers. Breathe in and out gently and deliberately and visualize the energy mounting where your middle fingers are pressed together.

33rd *Thing you need to know...*

The Sixth Step: Seishin Toitsu

Visualize the energy in your middle fingers moving to your root chakra each time you exhale. When you inhale, visualize the energy moving back into your fingertips. Avoid tracing the energy moving through your arms, your chest, and then down to your root chakra. Instead, focus on visualizing the energy passing immediately to the root chakra from your fingers and back again with each inhale and exhale. Perform this for about 5 minutes.

34th *Thing you need to know...*

The Seventh Step: Mokunen

Once the meditation is over and you feel calm and cleansed, then utter the words "I am now ending Hatsurei Ho." to seal the practice.

Keep in mind that this process of cleansing your energy and meditating isn't only beneficial in preparation for reiki healing. Finding time for this meditation process even when you don't intend to perform any healing can help keep your energy positive, and will help you maintain optimal wellness to prevent pent up negativity from building up inside your system.

35ᵗʰ Thing you need to know...

Refocus With Your Intention

As you go through the process of meditation, it would help to maintain or regain focus by reminding yourself of your intention. Repeat the intention to yourself like a mantra every so often to help keep your mind on the goal of your reiki healing session. If you have to, don't be afraid to word it out. Often, hearing the intention come from your own lips helps make it much more prominent in your mind.

36ᵗʰ Thing you need to know...

Activate Reiki Energy

During the meditation process, you should have been able to activate the reiki energy within yourself. If you feel like you need to heighten the energy even more, then you may need to follow a few more steps before you begin.

Hold your hands up to the sky with your palms facing upwards. Breathe deeply for a few minutes until you achieve a state of calm mindfulness. Visualize the positive ideas and feelings in your crown as an intense glow of bright, white light. Feel this energy travel down your head to your shoulders, arms, and finally to your hands.

Bring your hands slowly downwards and make them face each other, palm to palm, almost touching. Feel the warmth of the bright white healing energy as it grows between your palms. Hold the position for a few moments until you feel it's strong enough for healing.

Chapter 5: Basic Reiki Healing Techniques

Reiki healing practices are actually divided into three different lesson levels, each next level consisting of slightly more difficult concepts and techniques than the previous. For the purpose of this guide, we're going to focus on the most basic techniques to help you establish your practice and develop a deeper understanding of the foundations of reiki healing.

37th Thing you need to know...

Your Environment is Key

The efficacy of your reiki healing session will rely on how well you're able to focus your mind on the energy of reiki. If there are any distractions around you - such as physical discomfort, noise, or movement - then you might find it hard to maintain concentration on the task at hand.

For that reason, it's imperative that you optimize your environment to support your reiki healing practice. Here are some elements you might want to consider:

- Turn down the lights to a dim glow, as though you were preparing to sleep. Allowing just enough visibility so you can make your way around your space limits the distractions and visual stimulation you perceive during healing.

- Find a comfortable spot in your home. Be it a chair or your bed, make sure you're free from discomfort and pain, and that you can maintain your position in your chosen spot for the entire length of healing.

- Enhance the mood by lighting a few scented candles or by playing soothing music. The more relaxed and stress-free you feel, the more positive your energy becomes.

- Attend to all of your bodily needs. Drink water, relieve yourself, eat, and make sure you're well-rested before you start. Any bodily functions that get in the way of your healing can distract you from your goal and push you to cut your session short.

38th Thing you need to know...

Sense Your Body

The most basic aspect of the reiki healing technique is the process of *sensing your body*. The **full body scan** enables you to pick out different sensations throughout your body. The purpose of the scan is to determine where you should focus your healing energy.

This part of the process ties in with intention setting. If you want to use reiki healing for the purpose of *physical wellness*, then you may want to consider scanning your body before you set your intention. Doing so will help you target the areas that need the most attention.

Another benefit of the full body scan is that it enables you to reveal the truth of your life force. Not everyone is deeply attuned to their energy, and so it might be a challenge to fully understand when you're making an actual impact on your life force by way of reiki. Taking the time to 'sense' the energy in your body will help you attune to its properties and become more sensitive to changes, improvements, and blockages that it might manifest.

To start the full body scan, follow these steps:

- Lie down and try to achieve a state of mindfulness.

- Once in a mindful, meditative state, close your eyes and sense the toes on your feet. *How do they feel? Can you visualize the energy flowing through them? Do you sense any blockages?* Ask yourself these questions for each new part you progress to.

- Work your way slowly and deliberately from your feet, up to your knees, your thighs, until you reach the crown of your head. Always ask yourself the previous questions in order to properly investigate the status of the energy in that body part.

- Any areas where there might be a blockage should be remembered. Make a mental note of the parts of your body where you sense a potential disturbance.

- Throughout the process, *do not attempt to change anything*. If it happens that there's a blockage in a part of your body, don't attempt to release the tension just yet. The objective of the full body scan is not to heal but to help you understand where you should direct your healing energy.

39*th* Thing you need to know...
The Basic Reiki Hand Positions

There are an infinite number of hand positions in the reiki healing practice, each of which aims to target the different problems and ailments that people might experience. For this basic instruction, we're focusing on 15 different basic reiki hand positions that may come in handy as you learn the ropes.

These hand positions have no inherent meaning other than the fact that they aim to imbibe positive healing energy where it might be necessary. As the healer, it is up to you whether you feel more empowered when you touch the parts being addressed, or if you simply hover your hands over the target area. There is no right or wrong way.

- **Position 1** - Over the face with the fingers touching over the forehead

- **Position 2** - Over the head with fingers touching along the midline of the skull

- **Position 3** - Cupping the ears, with the fingers resting on the temples of the forehead

- **Position 4** - Along the nape, with the tips of the fingers touching gently

- **Position 5** - Over the shoulders, with the pinky side of the hand touching the neck

- **Position 6** - Just under the ribs, with the tips of the fingers touching

- **Position 7** - At the level of the belly button, fingers touching

- **Position 8** - At the level of the pubic bone, fingers touching

- **Position 9** - On the lower back just above the buttocks, fingers touching

- **Position 10** - Slightly higher on the lower back, over the sacral area, fingers touching

- **Position 11** - Bend down and hold the left foot with both hands

- **Position 12** - Bend down and hold the right foot with both hands

- **Position 13** - Bend down and hold the right foot with the right hand, and the left foot with the left hand simultaneously

40th Thing you need to know...

More Than Just Touching

These basic hand techniques don't only encourage you to touch your different body parts. There is a deep cognitive facet to these techniques, requiring the full participation of your mind and spirit in order to be truly effective in offering you healing.

During each step of the process, repeat your mantra and remind yourself *why* you're undergoing healing in the first place. Remember the areas of your body that piqued your interest during the full body scan that you performed prior to healing.

Every step of the way, try to maximize the feeling capabilities of your hands. *Focus on the healing energy passing through them.* Feel the warmth of your hands and visualize the energy in your system as you move along. In the areas of blockage, imaging the energy repairing damage and encouraging the ideal vibration and vigor where it might have been lost. Repeat to yourself, *"I am a child of the universe, and I deserve to heal."*

41st *Thing you need to know...*

The Possibilities are Endless

Even with these basic hand techniques, the possibilities of healing are endless. Using a combination of these hand gestures, or using them in sequence, can help you target a variety of problems. Remember, the key to an effective reiki healing practice *doesn't rely on how well you follow rules and sequences,* but on how well you're able to satisfy what feels right for your body.

42nd *Thing you need to know...*

There is No Single Right Way to Do It

Create your own healing sequences and follow what your body tells you. Be attuned with your system and truly *feel what your body needs*. The better you know your own body and the deeper you connect with your life force, the easier it becomes to use reiki healing.

Chapter 6:
Targeted Reiki Healing Sequences

If you're experiencing specific issues with your health or wellness, then you might want to target those particular problems to optimize the way you feel. While reiki is an art form that encourages you to be creative with your healing, there are certain patterns you can follow in order to address some of the more common wellness issues that people face.

43rd Thing you need to know...

Reiki Healing for Sleep

Having trouble falling asleep, staying asleep, or feeling satisfied after a long, night's sleep? There's a reiki healing sequence for that. After meditation and activating your reiki healing energy, focus on your crown.

Use **positions 1 to 4** and repeat your mantra for optimal sleep. Before moving on through the rest of the positions, cup your hands over your eyes, and say to yourself *"By this healing, I will achieve the most restful, satisfying sleep I've ever experienced."*

44ᵗʰ *Thing you need to know...*

Reiki Healing for Pain

Whether you had a nasty fall or if you just feel like your back is a little extra achy after slouching over your computer all day long, reiki can help you resolve physical, bodily pain to restore vigor and strength

Focus on the part of your body that's subject to pain. Visualize the blocked energy and focus your effort on enhancing the flow of life force through that area. See the pain as a red colored glow, slowly receding as you flood the area with your bright, white healing light.

45th *Thing you need to know...*

Reiki Healing for Stress

Stress is one of the major insults to our health. If you feel particularly stressed, take the time to relieve the tension and lift the pressure so that you can feel better prepared to face the challenges of your day to day life.

Position 5 typically works best for stress healing because it lifts the weight off of your shoulders and floods the body with positive healing energy. Take your time with position 5, spending between 15 to 30 minutes focusing on relieving stress. Visualize the negative energy being spun and shifted to a healthy, white glow that joins the positive healing energy emanating from your hands into your shoulders.

46th *Thing you need to know...*

Reiki Healing for Digestive Problems

Digestive problems can have significant impact

on your overall health because they also negatively affect your diet and nutrition. To target digestive problems, focus more on using the hand positions that focus on the abdomen and the lower back.

Take your time to feel and visualize the healing energy working through your system. Make sure you're using an intention that targets your digestive health. Visualize the negative energy in your digestive system being changed into positive, healing energy and imagine the toxins being cleansed from your body.

47th Thing you need to know...

Reiki Healing for Heartache

Maybe you went through a recent breakup, or maybe the relationship you had envisioned didn't pan out how you thought it would. When it comes to matters of the heart, reiki healing can offer significant benefits.

Set your intention to cleanse your mind and body of any negative emotions like sadness and grief. Claim that you will successfully move on from the heartache and find ew, true love in the not-so-distant future.

With your intention set, place your hands, one over the other, over the area of your heart. Visualize your healing energy enveloping your heart to overpower the negative emotions that exist therein. Let the energy flow through your body from your heart, taking with it any negativities and toxins that might have spread throughout your system.

At the end of the session, you should be able to visualize yourself glowing abundantly in white, healing energy.

48th Thing you need to know...
Reiki Healing for Financial Trouble

If you're going through financial trouble - as we all have - you might want to try this simple reiki healing technique for financial abundance. While seated comfortably in a chair, open up your palms to the heavens, stretching your arms out over your head.

Say something like, *"I am grateful for the abundance that the universe has graciously showered upon me and I claim more prosperity in the coming days."* Remember that gratefulness is a significant element of the reiki healing technique for financial stability.

Without gratefulness, we tend to feel negative towards what we have, thinking that *it isn't enough*. Instead of wrapping your head around the idea that you don't have enough money, try to change your perspective and be grateful for what it is that you already have. Then ask to receive more by the grace and charity of the universe around you.

49th Thing you need to know...

Reiki Healing for Your Career

It's not uncommon for us to feel dissatisfied with our work, especially if we've been doing it for a while. Healing your career is one of the many possibilities of reiki, allowing you to enjoy new found hope, vigor, and excitement for a job that might have been dragging you along for a while.

Place your hands together as if in prayer and imagine the white, healing light growing and glowing in between them. Feel the warmth in your hands and focus on the energy for a few minutes. Visualize the energy empowering your hands, and then place your hands on your head using the sequence of **positions 1 to 4**.

Express gratitude for the financial support that your career has given you through the years, and claim a fruitful, satisfying work life by the power of the universe around you. Envelope your mind in the healing energy of your hands, and visualize as it lifts the dissatisfaction away from your thoughts.

50th Thing you need to know...

Reiki Healing for the Common Cold

While doctors and scientists have yet to develop the cure for the common cold, reiki is a few steps ahead. The healing practice can help lift the symptoms of the cold and flu, enabling you to resume your usual activities and work without the discomfort caused by these common illnesses.

During the basic healing sequence, visualize the viral infection as a glowing, negative energy throughout your system. As you impart healing energy with your touch, visualize it wrapping around the negative energy to create more healing power. Imagine the negative energy being cleansed away as your healing energy passes through the different parts of your body.

51st Thing you need to know...

Reiki Healing for Allergies and Congestion

Allergic reactions can sap your energy and make you feel unproductive. But with the right reiki healing technique, you can dial down the effects of allergies and breathe more freely to support your everyday activities.

Hold your hands one over the other over your chest. Breathe in and out deliberately and slowly and visualize your lungs inflating and deflating with each breath. If your nose is too congested to breathe through, breathe in and out through puckered lips.

Envision the healing energy growing in your chest with each new breath. Feel the congestion and irritation being eased away with revived life force and visualize the negativity and toxins being lifted from your system.

Chapter 7:
Healing Others with
Reiki

The beauty of reiki is that aside from enabling you to target your own energy flaws, the process also teaches you how to address possible energy problems that other people are experiencing. The ancient healing art was developed for you to be able to *share* your enlightenment, spreading positivity and good vibrations to others around you.

52nd *Thing you need to know…*

It Starts the Same Way

When healing another person with reiki, the entire process starts the same way. That is, you meditate together using the Hatsurei Ho method. Give your participant a few short instructions to give them the basics of the meditative process. Try to achieve a state of mindful calm together and ask them to break their own limitations before the start of the process.

53ʳᵈ Thing you need to know...

It Won't Work with Doubt

If your participant feels doubtful at any point of the process, then it's possible that you might not achieve a fruitful session. Remember, reiki healing will only be as effective as you believe it to be. Before you start, ask your participant if they have any apprehensions and doubts. Try to break through the doubt by asking them to write down their own affirmations.

54ᵗʰ Thing you need to know...

Brainstorm an Intention

What does your participant want to achieve? Why did they ask you for assistance? Remember, the intention will always have to come from the person being healed, and not from you. So, if for instance, you're working on a friend and you've noticed that they've been struggling with a specific issue, don't suggest an intention for them.

Instead, ask them questions that encourage them to really assess their own personal situation. *"What aspect of your daily life are you experiencing the most difficulty with?", "Is there anything in particular that's making you feel negatively about yourself or others?", "What part of your life do you want to improve the most?", "Are there any physical aches, pains, or illness that you want to address today?"*

Remind your participant that the objective is to heal him or herself. Intentions that involve other people in their lives might not be ideal. Teach the basics of intention setting and guide your participant towards the right phrasing.

55ᵗʰ *Thing you need to know...*
Prepare for the Healing Process

Ask your participant to get comfortable. They can be seated or they can lie down, depending on what feels most ideal for them. One of the benefits of reiki healing is that it doesn't require participants to wear a certain type of clothing or to be bare during the process.

If you're participant is wearing layered clothing, like a jacket or sweater on top of a shirt, then you can ask them to remove the outermost layer of clothing. But other than that, participants can remain fully clothed.

Before you start the session, ask your participant whether they would be more comfortable receiving direct touch or if they'd prefer to have your hands hover over their body instead. Some people who might be new to the process of reiki healing may prefer that you keep your hands at a slight distance.

56th Thing you need to know...

Activating Your Healing Power

Now that your participant is ready and their intention is made clear, it's time to activate your healing power. In the same process as you would during self-healing, raise your hands to the sky, palm side up. Visualize positive healing energy glowing in your hands, traveling down to your heart and through your entire body.

Say, *"I am endowed with the healing power of the universe. Let me hands impart nothing but light, love, and positive vibrations."*

Once you feel the full warmth of your healing energy emanating from your hands, start the hand placement process in the same sequence described for self-healing. Start from the head, working your way down towards the feet. Be sure to take more time over the areas of the body associated with your participant's intention.

57th *Thing you need to know...*

Healing Remotely

More experienced reiki healers can actually send their healing efforts from a remote location, enabling them to touch the lives and tap into the life force of individuals from miles away. Performed similarly to the healing technique described above, **distance healing** can have the same impact. The difference is that the healer and the participant aren't in the same room.

The distance healing technique is often taught in greater detail to individuals receiving instruction for Reiki II. The process requires quite a bit of practice and an in-depth attunement with your own personal healing energy. Nonetheless, it can be an effective way to heal others who might not be in your immediate presence.

58th Thing you need to know...

Sealing the Healing Session

At the end of the healing session, it's important that you seal the process that took place. Sealing the healing session sets the positive energy in place and cleanses away any remaining toxicity or negativity in the space.

To seal your session, simply hold your hands together as if in prayer. Offer gratitude for the opportunity to provide healing to others around you, and give thanks to your participant for trusting you with the experience. If you feel it's necessary - especially if you had to deal with heavy emotions during the healing - cleanse your hands and the space with a clear quartz stone.

59th Thing you need to know...

Reiki Healing Doesn't Have to Be a Standalone Technique

Again, reiki isn't tied to any belief system or religion, so it's possible for you to use it in conjunction with a variety of other techniques used for spiritual and holistic healing. Creating the ideal combination of steps and strategies can help you establish a practice that's truly fulfilling and satisfying for you and those seeking your healing energy.

Chapter 8:
Reiki Healing and
Other Disciplines

Reiki healing is the ideal component to add to a holistic healing practice because it fits well with a variety of other techniques. The process can be tied into a list of other mystic arts in order to achieve full body wellness like never before.

60th Thing you need to know...

Crystal Healing

Crystal healing is the practice of harnessing the power of naturally occurring crystals. Each type of crystal offers a unique benefit, and they all resonate with *perfect vibrations* that work to optimize the flow of energy throughout our systems.

61st *Thing you need to know...*

Combining Reiki with Crystals

Reiki healing and the use of crystals can tie in closely to one another because of the similarities in their purpose and the way that they tend to complement one another. The purpose of reiki healing is to optimize the flow of life force by using healing energy to remove negativity and blockage. In the same way, the use of crystals is said to relieve negative energy forces and blockages in a person's system.

There are a number of ways that you can incorporate crystals into your reiki healing practice. And by evolving your technique to incorporate the mystical healing properties of these natural stones, you can achieve healing to a far greater extent.

62nd *Thing you need to know...*

Cleansing Before and After Reiki Healing

Remember that one of the essential aspects of an effective reiki healing session is the environment where you intend to perform the practice. If there are negative energy vibrations in the space, then these might interfere with your healing session.

To start, always use a clear crystal quartz point to clean away any negative energies in your space. In the same way, you may also want to clean the area after the reiki healing session. Using the same kind of stone after your practice can remove any negative energy which was lifted from you or your participant during the healing session from the area.

63rd Thing you need to know...
Reiki Healing with Crystals

Crystals can be used for healing in a variety of ways, including pendulum swinging and placing. These methods overlap with the reiki healing techniques, making it an intuitive option for those who want to maximize the benefits of their healing practice.

During the process of reiki healing, choose a crystal that works well with your intention or the intention of your participant. Hold the stone in your hand using your thumb, pressing the stone into your palm.

Make sure the rest of your fingers are open to allow your own healing energy to pass through. Go on through the process using the same technique, the main difference being the presence of the stone in your hands. Feel its power strengthening your own healing energy as you move your hands over the different parts of the body.

64th *Thing you need to know...*

Meditating with Crystals

The more attuned you are with your healing energy, the more effective your healing practice becomes. Clearing away negative vibrations by using crystals can help you hone your healing capabilities and become a more effective reiki healer.

During Hatsurei Ho, try to use a crystal or two to hold in your palm while you meditate. This should help you receive their positive vibrations to achieve a deeper connection with your inner healing potential.

65th *Thing you need to know...*

Creating a Grid

Crystal grids are layouts that are designed to resonate vibrations in an effort to achieve a specific goal or intention. Creating a grid to resonate with positive energy can make you feel more connected with your inner healer. Try forming a crystal pattern in the space where you often perform reiki healing. Set the invention of maximizing your healing energy so as to improve the outcomes of your reiki practice.

66th Thing you need to know...

Chakra Healing

Chakra healing is an ancient healing art form that focuses on chakras - energy vortexes in our bodies where life force tends to collect. These intersections of energy each represent a unique function, purpose, or quality that we possess. Any problems in the flow of energy through these energy centers can result in a diverse range of problems involving our physical, emotional, mental, or sexual well-being .

67th Thing you need to know...

Combining Reiki Healing and Chakra Principles

It is possible to use reiki in combination with chakra principles. Essentially, chakra healing tells us that there are *specific, localized, standardized* areas in the body where *energy centers exist.* By directing our reiki healing efforts to these chakras, we can optimize their flow and relieve the symptoms of poor life force. During the reiki healing process, simple target the chakras using your hand placing techniques. Maintain focus on the chakra and visualize the energy center spinning and glowing as you impart your healing energy.

68th *Thing you need to know...*

Targeting Your Chakras

There are 7 main chakras in the traditional chakra system, and each one corresponds to different body parts, symptoms, problems, and aspects of your life. Understanding how each one works will help you better pinpoint which chakra to target during your healing practice in order to achieve your intention.

The 7 main chakras extend along the length of the spine, so it might be hard to place your own hands over them during the reiki healing process. Instead, place your hands over your chest, abdomen, and pelvis in order to direct healing energy towards your energy centers. Visualize each center as you do so in order to positively impact them through reiki healing.

69th *Thing you need to know…*

Yoga

Yoga is a movement healing practice that aims to restore proper energy flow and balance by moving the physical body. It's believed that through yoga, participants can connect with their spiritual self in order to achieve optimal wellness between mind, body, and spirit.

70th *Thing you need to know…*

Combining Yoga and Reiki Healing

The process of combining yoga with reiki healing can be slightly more complicated than the previous two because there will be technical knowledge necessary. It's important that you first have a steady foundation in both practices before you're able to reap the full benefits of their combined power.

In essence however, reiki and yoga go together by incorporating the hand placement techniques for reiki into the many different postures and poses in the yoga practice. *Swiping* the hands over certain body parts as you transition from one pose to another can help improve the healing process, allowing you to impart more healing energy to areas of your body that might need it.

Chapter 9:
Reiki Symbols and
Their Meanings

One of the principles you're likely to encounter as you learn more about reiki is that the practice uses a range of *symbols*. These written codes are said to guide students who hope to learn and hone their reiki healing capabilities. Keep in mind that the symbols themselves do not hold any unique power. Instead, it's the user who imbibes power into the symbols to make them beneficial during the practice of reiki.

71st Thing you need to know...

Understanding How to Use Reiki Symbols

Reiki symbols are not charged with any energy, and they actually don't have any power over the user at any point in the process. So, you can't merely scribble the symbol on a slip of paper and hope that it magically casts its effects onto you.

Instead, think of the symbols as visual guides. The more often you see them, the stronger their associations become. Creating a strong connection in your mind between these symbols and the properties they symbolize can make it easier for you as a healer to tap into the healing energy needed to produce the outcomes that the symbols represent.

72ⁿᵈ *Thing you need to know...*

There are Five Basic Reiki Symbols

Level II reiki healers will know at least five basic reiki symbols. These were traditionally taught by Usui himself, and are said to have been part of the visions he experienced when he had his spiritual awakening. Each symbol represents a specific quality or purpose, and thus they become relevant depending on the intention you wish to set.

73rd Thing you need to know...

The Power Reiki Symbol

Represented by a coil, the Power Reiki symbol otherwise known Cho Ku Rei, is the symbol for the power of the universe. The symbol is most often used at the start and end of a healing session to boost your abilities and give you more potent healing capabilities to start and end your practice.

74th Thing you need to know...

The Mental and Emotional Reiki Symbol

Also sometimes called the Harmony symbol, the Sei Hei Ki symbol is used to represent the balance between the mind and body. The Japanese name for the symbol literally translates to "God and man become one." During healing, the symbol finds its role as a grounding energy. It releases deep-seated negative energy and casts it out from the body.

75th Thing you need to know...
The Distance Reiki Symbol

In traditional Usui teaching, the Distance Reiki symbol is called Hon Sha Ze Sho Nen. When translated, that means "having no present, past, or future." In essence, this symbol can be called upon to heal the problems of the past, the present, and the possible problems of the future. Instead of simply using it during the reiki healing practice, you can also call in this symbol during your day to day life to reap its benefits.

76th Thing you need to know...
The Master Reiki Symbol

This symbol generally means 'great enlightenment' when translated from its Japanese name 'Da Ko Myo', and is often considered the most powerful of all. It combines the powers of the first three symbols and is rarely called upon. That's because its energy is used specifically to enhance the overall benefits of reiki and every other form of healing that you might seek out to optimize your health and wellness.

77th Thing you need to know...

The Completion Reiki Symbol

Also called Raku in Japanese, the Completion Reiki symbol grounds and seals new found reiki healing energy. The symbol for Raku resembles a lightning bolt and symbolizes the energy or life force that flows down our spine. It is believed that Raku was not originally taught by Usui, but it has found its place among the four traditional symbols. It's called upon to set positive energy in place and prevent it from being corrupted.

78th Thing you need to know...

Calling on the Symbols of Reiki During Healing

One of the ways that you can use these reiki symbols is by calling them during the healing process. Studying each symbol, remembering how they're written or drawn, and associating them with their intended purpose can make it easier to call on their benefits when you need them.

For instance, if you're going through the process of self-healing and you sense that there's a disturbance in the strength of your life force in the area of your chest, then you can visualize the power reiki symbol to reap its advantages and strengthen the flow of energy in the area you want to address.

79ᵗʰ *Thing you need to know...*

Sending Healing Vibrations with Symbols

If for instance, you have a friend or family member who says they're dealing with illness, you can help them heal by sending them positive vibrations through the use of reiki symbols. Visualize each symbol one by one and repeat their Japanese names as you think of their associated symbol.

Repeat each one in a cycle and envision the person you want to send positive vibrations to.

Then as the power of your healing energy mounts, cast it out towards the universe, and direct it to the person you want to help. It may also help to say their name before you release the energy, and to focus on their image by looking at a picture of them as you build your energy and your intention.

80th Thing you need to know...

Sending Reiki to a Future Event

There might be times that you feel apprehensive about a future event, like a doctor's appointment or a job interview. If you want to feel calm and at peace on that significant event in your life, then you might want to send reiki to that future date.

Chant the names of the first three symbols and visualize yourself on the day that you're focusing on. Imagine the way you would want to act or feel on the day and claim that you will succeed and you will receive blessings on that day. Once you fully envelope your mind around that thought, absorb the positive healing energy you've mounted and say, *"By the power of the universe, I will overcome my apprehension and see prosperity on that day."*

81ˢᵗ *Thing you need to know...*

Strengthening an Intention

If you like writing down your intention, then you might also want to incorporate the use of symbols. As you read your intention to yourself, draw the five symbols of reiki around it. Draw as many as you want and visualize the purpose they represent. Feel your intention charging with positive energy and then ground yourself in their vibrations by chanting "*Sei Hei Ki.*"

Chapter 10:
Tips to Maximize Your Reiki Healing Practice

We all stumble and we all question our technique at some point. It's only natural to wonder whether you're doing the right thing - that only means that you care about the outcomes of your practice. Make sure you keep these tips in mind when you perform self-healing or if you try to heal others around you to maximize the benefits that you take from the experience.

82nd *Thing you need to know...*
Go With Your Gut

A lot of people tend to feel confused with spiritual healing methods like reiki or crystal healing because there isn't a clear, step-by-step procedure. Methods change and that tends to confuse beginners. But the reason why you might find different people doing different things is because *there isn't a single way to do things.*

In essence, you should follow your gut. *If it feels right, it probably is.* Your body and spirit will know better than your mind because your thoughts tend to be tainted with external influences around you and doubt. If all else fails, close your eyes and sense your body. It will tell you what to do.

83ʳᵈ *Thing you need to know...*

Experiment Freely

Hand placement techniques aren't set in stone. In the same way that you should trust your gut when it comes to the process of reiki healing, you should also follow your gut when it comes to hand placement.

Experiment with different hand placement positions and techniques. As long as you're using positive energy and your intentions are pure, there will be a benefit to the strategy you choose.

84th Thing you need to know...

Practice Frequently

The principle "practice makes perfect" is most true when applied to reiki healing. That's because the more you try, the deeper your connection with your healing energy becomes. Remember - not everyone is aware of their unique capabilities to heal themselves and others around them. By continued practice, you can establish a stronger connection with your own talents.

85th Thing you need to know...

Hone Your Sensitivity

Many of us end up overlooking the effects of reiki healing, watering down our satisfaction because our expectations were not met. But sometimes, it just takes a stronger sensitivity to change in order to see the benefits of the process. Understand that reiki healing *will likely not produce significant leaps and bounds of change in your life*. The differences may be subtle, but with continued practice, you can discover a greater sense of satisfaction in the process and what it brings to your life.

86th Thing you need to know...

Set Reasonable Intentions

Another reason why some people feel unhappy with their reiki healing results is because they set intentions that were too impractical, unattainable, or even questionable in terms of positivity. For instance, setting the intention *"I will lose 100 pounds within the next 2 months to spite my ex for leaving me"* doesn't sound like a very good intention, now does it?

Always be positive with your intentions and never aim to bear ill will to anyone around you. Remember, you are the focus of your healing and not anyone else. Plus, it pays to keep your intentions within logical limits. While it is possible to lose weight with reiki, it won't happen in a snap. Instead of asking for results, ask for the discipline and motivation to achieve the body you want.

87th Thing you need to know…
Optimize Your Life

Reiki is a *holistic* healing process, so it's only expected that you involve your entire being in the process. It's not enough to ask the universe for healing and then wait for it to do everything on its own while you sit back and reap the benefits. No, reiki teaches you to be *a part of your own healing*.

Use reiki to help you establish healthy eating habits, exercise routines, and self-care patterns. Aim to optimize your *entire being* in order to fully appreciate the healing benefits of reiki.

88th *Thing you need to know...*

Don't Rely on Yourself

It's easy to get lost in the idea that you're a great healer when there are lots of people seeking your help. But don't let the clamor for your healing energy get he best of you. There is power in humility.

The moment you start to believe that you're responsible for the healing that other people experience, that's when you start to adapt negativity into your life. Remember that *you* are not the one healing others, but the positive reiki energy that flows *through you*. We are merely vessels that demonstrate the healing power of the universe and we are not directly responsible for the relief that other people feel.

89th *Thing you need to know...*

Cast Out Negative Energy

One of the most common mistakes that beginners make when performing reiki healing is forgetting to cast out negative energy. When you heal yourself, you release negativity that was once a part of your system. Allowing that to stay in your environment could mean that the same negativity could attack your system in the future.

Don't forget to cleanse your space to cast negative energy out into the universe and away from your space. You can do this by using crystal grids or by basking your space in sage smoke.

90th *Thing you need to know...*

Adapt a Mindful Lifestyle

When you start to open up your healing energy to the universe, you'll become more aware of the things happening around you. Sometimes, it will take a cerebral effort to fully adapt a mindful lifestyle after your reiki healing has opened up your potential.

Be aware of the way that you respond to people and situations around you. Make an effort to consciously avoid negative reactions like anger, guilt, sadness, and disappointment. There are *always better ways* to react to the things that happen around you. *You* are in control of your own self. Don't let people or situations cause you to invite negativity into your life.

91st *Thing you need to know...*

Use It Daily

Reiki is best appreciated as a daily solution against the many different issues that we face. Performing a healing session at least once a day can help you maximize the benefits of the process and truly enjoy the advantages it brings. Some people do this by performing reiki healing right before they hop out of bed to start the day.

But reiki doesn't stop with the healing process itself. Aim to adapt a reiki healing mindset throughout the day. Focus on your healing energy whenever you find some spare time and release negativity whenever you can to avoid having it build up inside you.

Chapter 11:
The Effects of Reiki Healing

Aside from the benefits that reiki brings in relation to the intention you set, there are other markers of the practice taking form in your life. By picking out these manifestations, you'll see just how powerful reiki can be as a healing tool for holistic wellness in your life.

92nd *Thing you need to know...*

You'll Feel an Abundance of Energy

You'll wake up feeling energetic, like you have more power to spend on the different things you need to do. You'll feel vigor and excitement like never before, like you're ready and willing to face the challenges that lie ahead. Even when all of your obligations have been completed, you'll find that you have power to perform *more* and to try new things.

93rd *Thing you need to know...*
You'll Be More Intuitive with Relationships

When you release your reiki healing potential, you become more attuned to the feelings that other people might experience. That's because as a healer, sensitivity becomes one of your most powerful qualities.

When you interact with people, you become more aware of how to act, how to respond, and how to approach them because you understand how they feel. This makes you more effective in handling your relationships, enabling you to achieve more satisfying, less confrontational communication and contact with the key people in your life.

94th *Thing you need to know...*
You'll Be Less Bothered

The more you practice reiki healing, the more valuable your peace becomes. You will learn to protect it at all costs. One of the things you'll notice is that you might feel far less affected when people or situations don't turn out how you want them to. You'll be more mature when it comes to handling frustrating instances, and you'll be far less likely to spend your energy thinking about things that would have otherwise made you feel upset.

95th *Thing you need to know...*
You'll Feel Healthier

Your energy ties in with your physical health. The more efficiently your energy moves through your body, the less prone to physical stress and injury you'll become. With frequent reiki healing, you might find yourself feeling stronger and more capable of fighting off illness, if it even comes at all. With your optimal energy flow, you'll be better equipped to face infection and disease without fully succumbing to their effects.

96th *Thing you need to know...*
You'll Move On Easier

There are just some things that are hard to let go. An old friend that betrayed you, family members who didn't see your worth, an abusive boss that might have caused you to lose opportunities for your career in the past.

While it might be hard to let these things go, opening your reiki healing potential will make it possible for you to release pent up negativity from the past. As you continue your healing practice, you'll find yourself more capable and willing to release past events that you might have held on to throughout the years because of a new found sense of peace.

97th Thing you need to know...

You'll Rest and Relax Effortlessly

In the past, you might have found yourself lying in bed for hours, tossing and turning as you try to fall asleep. But after reiki healing, you might fall asleep effortlessly each night. The release of negative energy puts your mind, body, and soul at peace. With far less to think about during the night, you can enjoy more restful sleep that rewards you with renewed health and vigor with each new day.

98th Thing you need to know...

You'll Achieve Optimal Work-Life Balance

If you used to feel overloaded with all of the different responsibilities and obligations of adult life, reiki healing will help you achieve optimal work-life balance. The proper flow of energy helps you to map out your own capabilities. Giving you a deep sense of peace, reiki can clear your mind of clutter and thoughts, and give you a more intuitive, practical train of thought that puts things into proper perspective to achieve optimal balance.

99th Thing you need to know...

You'll Feel Fresher and Pain-Free

Maybe you used to struggle with chronic back pain. We've all been there. But reiki is a powerful solution to combat those aches and pains. Optimizing the flow of life force through these injured parts of your system, reiki improves your body's resistance to pain and helps damaged tissues heal more rapidly.

100th Thing you need to know...

You'll Feel Spiritually Richer

Not everyone has a deep connection with their spirituality because it exists on a plane that's not tangible to the five senses. But with reiki, you'll achieve a much deeper understanding of your own spirituality and faith. Connecting with the universe enriches the soul and may even give you an insight on deeper truths that might not have been clear to you before.

101st *Thing you need to know…*

You'll Be Protected From Future Insult

Just like a car that's routinely maintained and tuned-up, or a race horse that's fed and trained for optimal performance, your energy flow also requires regular care. With frequent reiki healing, you can prevent negative energy from building up inside your system and wreaking significant damage later on.

Performing reiki healing *today* protects you from insult *tomorrow,* making you better prepared to face the world around you and the unexpected things that tomorrow might bring.

Conclusion

In our modern world, it's easy to *settle for a quality of life that doesn't truly meet our expectations*. We're always tired, we're always working, and we're never happy - but we continue on because we think that this is how life is supposed to be.

But thanks to people like Dr. Usui, more and more of us are learning that life doesn't have to be unsatisfying. You can be happy, you can have that vigor for life coursing through your veins, and you can experience day to day life on a higher level than ever before. It all depends on how well you can tap into your own healing potential.

The power to heal and optimize your life lies within your own hands - you only need to discover and activate it to make a change in the way you experience day to day events. In fact, you might just even be the vessel the universe is waiting for in order to impart valuable positive energy to the people around you.

So, don't let your healing potential stay

stagnant and go to waste. Awaken the mystic healer within and discover just how you can be the answer to the pains and dissatisfaction you might experience with life. Tap into the reiki healer within and experience the fullness of the universe's positivity coursing through your life.

It's all in your hands.

Made in the USA
Monee, IL
12 May 2020